The New Renal Diet Cookbook

How to Control Your Weight and Start a New and Better Lifestyle. Eating Healthier and Tastier With the Most Complete Collection of Renal Diet Recipes

Karen Perry

TABLE OF CONTENTS

INTRODUCTION

Nothing can surpass vegetarian foods to keep your kidneys healthy, and I'm a big fan of plant-based weight loss diets. I was lucky that my wife passed it on to me because the natural weight loss pills were too short at the time. Fortunately, it was eventually wound up by a healthy diet of fruits, vegetables, nuts and seeds sprinkled with salt.

The following recipes for healthy kidney nutrition are suitable for people with kidney disease, as they are free of foods that promote inflammation and other problems. Here is an overview of kidney nutrition and guidelines, and talk to someone familiar with their own kidney disease to find a meal plan that works for you. The following recipe for healthy kidney nutrition is suitable for people without kidney disease, as it is free of foods that promote inflammatory bowel disease, diabetes, high blood pressure, high blood pressure or other health problems. It is also appropriate for someone with kidney disease and / or kidney failure to talk to your doctor or dietitian or someone in your health care system about what meals are appropriate for them and their diet.

If you suffer from kidney disease or are on kidney dialysis, you must follow a kidney dietary plan. If you have kidney disease or kidney failure, you should include the following information on kidney nutrition and guidelines for healthy kidney nutrition in your diet so that, even if you intend to follow a healthy kidney nutrition plan, as a first step, you can equip your kitchen with the right foods.

A kidney diet or diet plan, also known as kidney disease, limits the intake of sodium, potassium, and phosphorus because people with kidney disease or kidney problems must monitor how much of these nutrients they consume. It is a weight loss diet, but it is also a dietary plan for kidney health, especially those that limit the intake of sodium and potassium (phosphorus). A kidney diet or diet plan, also known as a kidney disease diet, restricts the intake of sodium, potassium or phosphorus, as people with kidney diseases such as kidney cancer, kidney failure, kidney failure and kidney dialysis cannot consume the same nutrients as normal people.

Basically, a kidney diet is a way of eating that helps protect the kidneys from further damage, and it is also a weight loss diet for kidney health.

If you eat right and incorporate physical activity into your routine, you will lose unwanted pounds, feel healthier, lose weight and feel better. When you work with a kidney dietitian, your diet will help you avoid heart disease, diabetes, high blood pressure, weakened bones, kidney disease and other health problems.

It is a good Mediterranean diet pill and holds back the negative effects of a diet for a while. Tea weight loss surgery helps with weight loss, but you can run away from it by taking a Soldier's Corn pill. It helps to drive away enemies who have attacked you before and helps to drive away the attack.

BREAKFAST

1. Pasta with Indian Lentils

Preparation Time: 5 minutes

Cooking Time: 0 minutes

Servings: 6

Ingredients:

- ¼-½ cup fresh cilantro (chopped)
- 3 cups water
- 2 small dry red peppers (whole)
- 1 teaspoon turmeric
- 1 teaspoon ground cumin
- 2-3 cloves garlic (minced)
- 1 can (15 ounces) cubed Red bell peppers (with juice)
- 1 large onion (chopped)
- ½ cup dry lentils (rinsed)
- ½ cup orzo or tiny pasta

Directions:

1. In a skillet, combine all ingredients except for the cilantro then boil on medium-high heat.
2. Ensure to cover and slightly reduce heat to medium-low and simmer until pasta is tender for about 35 minutes.

3. Afterwards, take out the chili peppers then add cilantro and top it with low-fat sour cream.

Nutrition: Calories: 175; Carbs: 40g; Protein: 3g; Fats: 2g; Phosphorus: 139mg; Potassium: 513mg; Sodium: 61mg

2. Pineapple Bread

Preparation Time: 20 Minutes

Cooking Time: 1 Hour

Servings: 10

Ingredients:

- 1/3 cup Swerve
- 1/3 cup butter, unsalted
- 2 eggs
- 2 cups flour
- 3 teaspoons baking powder
- 1 cup pineapple, undrained
- 6 cherries, chopped

Directions:

1. Whisk the Swerve with the butter in a mixer until fluffy.
2. Stir in the eggs, then beat again.
3. Add the baking powder and flour, then mix well until smooth.
4. Fold in the cherries and pineapple.
5. Spread this cherry-pineapple batter in a 9x5 inch baking pan.
6. Bake the pineapple batter for 1 hour at 350 degrees F.
7. Slice the bread and serve.

Nutrition: Calories 197, Total Fat 7.2g, Sodium 85mg, Dietary Fiber 1.1g, Sugars 3 g, Protein 4g, Calcium 79mg, Phosphorous 316mg, Potassium 227mg

3. Parmesan Zucchini Frittata

Preparation Time: 10 minutes

Cooking Time: 35 minutes

Servings: 6

Ingredients:

- 1 tablespoon olive oil
- 1 cup yellow onion, sliced
- 3 cups zucchini, chopped
- ½ cup Parmesan cheese, grated
- 8 large eggs
- 1/2 teaspoon black pepper
- 1/8 teaspoon paprika
- 3 tablespoons parsley, chopped

Directions:

1. Toss the zucchinis with the onion, parsley, and all other ingredients in a large bowl.
2. Pour this zucchini-garlic mixture in an 11x7 inches pan and spread it evenly.
3. Bake the zucchini casserole for approximately 35 minutes at 350 degrees F.
4. Cut in slices and serve.

Nutrition: Calories 142, Total Fat 9.7g, Saturated Fat 2.8g, Cholesterol 250mg Sodium 123mg, Carbohydrate 4.7g, Dietary Fiber 1.3g, Sugars 2.4g, Protein 10.2g, Calcium 73mg, Phosphorous 375mg, Potassium 286mg

4. Garlic Mayo Bread

Preparation Time: 10 minutes

Cooking Time: 5 minutes

Servings: 16

Ingredients:

- 3 tablespoons vegetable oil
- 4 cloves garlic, minced
- 2 teaspoons paprika
- Dash cayenne pepper
- 1 teaspoon lemon juice
- 2 tablespoons Parmesan cheese, grated
- 3/4 cup mayonnaise
- 1 loaf (1 lb.) French bread, sliced
- 1 teaspoon Italian herbs

Directions:

1. Mix the garlic with the oil in a small bowl and leave it overnight.
2. Discard the garlic from the bowl and keep the garlic-infused oil.
3. Mix the garlic-oil with cayenne, paprika, lemon juice, mayonnaise, and Parmesan.
4. Place the bread slices in a baking tray lined with parchment paper.

5. Top these slices with the mayonnaise mixture and drizzle the Italian herbs on top.

6. Broil these slices for 5 minutes until golden brown.

7. Serve warm.

Nutrition: Calories 217, Total Fat 7.9g, Sodium 423mg, Dietary Fiber 1.3g, Sugars 2g, Protein 7g, Calcium 56mg, Phosphorous 347mg, Potassium 72mg

5. Strawberry Topped Waffles

Preparation Time: 15 minutes

Cooking Time: 20 minutes

Servings: 5

Ingredients:

- 1 cup flour
- 1/4 cup Swerve
- 1 ¾ teaspoons baking powder
- 1 egg, separated
- ¾ cup almond milk
- ½ cup butter, melted
- ½ teaspoon vanilla extract
- Fresh strawberries, sliced

Directions:

1. Prepare and preheat your waffle pan following the instructions of the machine.
2. Begin by mixing the flour with Swerve and baking soda in a bowl.
3. Separate the egg yolks from the egg whites, keeping them in two separate bowls.
4. Add the almond milk and vanilla extract to the egg yolks.
5. Stir the melted butter and mix well until smooth.

6. Now beat the egg whites with an electric beater until foamy and fluffy.

7. Fold this fluffy composition in the egg yolk mixture.

8. Mix it gently until smooth, then add in the flour mixture.

9. Stir again to make a smooth mixture.

10. Pour a half cup of the waffle batter in a preheated pan and cook until the waffle is done.

11. Cook more waffles with the remaining batter.

12. Serve fresh with strawberries on top.

Nutrition: Calories 342, Total Fat 20.5g,Sodium 156mg, Dietary Fiber 0.7g, Sugars 3.5g, Protein 4.8g, Calcium 107mg, Phosphorous 126mg, Potassium 233mg

6. Cheese Spaghetti Frittata

Preparation Time: 10 minutes

Cooking Time: 10 minutes

Servings: 6

Ingredients:

- 4 cups whole-wheat spaghetti, cooked
- 4 teaspoons olive oil
- 3 medium onions, chopped
- 4 large eggs
- 1/2 cup almond milk
- 1/3 cup Parmesan cheese, grated
- 2 tablespoons fresh parsley, chopped
- 2 tablespoons fresh basil, chopped
- 1/2 teaspoon black pepper
- 1 tomato, diced

Directions:

1. Set a suitable non-stick skillet over moderate heat and add in the olive oil.
2. Place the spaghetti in the skillet and cook by stirring for 2 minutes on moderate heat.
3. Whisk the eggs with almond milk, parsley, and black pepper in a bowl.

4. Pour this almond milky egg mixture over the spaghetti and top it all with basil, cheese, and tomato.

5. Cover the spaghetti frittata again with a lid and cook for approximately 8 minutes on low heat.

6. Slice and serve.

Nutrition: Calories 230, Total Fat 7.8g, Sodium 77mg, Dietary Fiber 5.6g, Sugars 4.5g, Protein 11.1g, Calcium 88mg, Phosphorous 368 mg, Potassium 214mg,

7. Shrimp Bruschetta

Preparation Time: 15 minutes

Cooking Time: 10 minutes

Servings: 4

Ingredients:

- 13 oz. shrimps, peeled
- 1 tablespoon tomato sauce
- ½ teaspoon Splenda
- ¼ teaspoon garlic powder
- 1 teaspoon fresh parsley, chopped
- ½ teaspoon olive oil
- 1 teaspoon lemon juice
- 4 whole-grain bread slices
- 1 cup water, for cooking

Directions:

1. In the saucepan, pour water and bring it to boil.
2. Add shrimps and boil them over the high heat for 5 minutes.
3. After this, drain shrimps and chill them to the room temperature.
4. Mix up together shrimps with Splenda, garlic powder, tomato sauce, and fresh parsley.
5. Add lemon juice and stir gently.

6. Preheat the oven to 360f.

7. Coat the slice of bread with olive oil and bake for 3 minutes.

8. Then place the shrimp mixture on the bread. Bruschetta is cooked.

Nutrition: Calories 199, Fat 3.7, Fiber 2.1, Carbs 15.3, Protein 24.1 Calcium 79mg, Phosphorous 316mg, Potassium 227mg Sodium: 121 mg

LUNCH

8. Marinated Shrimp Pasta Salad

Preparation Time: 15 minutes

Cooking Time: 5 hours

Servings: 1

Ingredients:

- 1/4 cup of honey
- 1/4 cup of balsamic vinegar
- 1/2 of an English cucumber, cubed
- 1/2 pound of fully cooked shrimp
- 15 baby carrots
- 1.5 cups of dime-sized cut cauliflower
- 4 stalks of celery, diced
- 1/2 large yellow bell pepper (diced)
- 1/2 red onion (diced)
- 1/2 large red bell pepper (diced)
- 12 ounces of uncooked tri-color pasta (cooked)
- 3/4 cup of olive oil
- 3 tsp. of mustard (Dijon)
- 1/2 tsp. of garlic (powder)
- 1/2 tsp. pepper

Directions:

1. Cut vegetables and put them in a bowl with the shrimp.

2. Whisk together the honey, balsamic vinegar, garlic powder, pepper, and Dijon mustard in a small bowl. While still whisking, slowly add the oil and whisk it all together.

3. Add the cooked pasta to the bowl with the shrimp and vegetables and mix it.

4. Toss the sauce to coat the pasta, shrimp, and vegetables evenly.

5. Cover and chill for a minimum of five hours before serving. Stir and serve while chilled.

Nutrition: Calories: 205 Fat: 13g Carbs: 10g Protein: 12g Sodium: 363mg Potassium: 156mg Phosphorus: 109mg

9. Peanut Butter and Jelly Grilled Sandwich

Preparation Time: 5 minutes

Cooking Time: 5 minutes

Servings: 1

Ingredients:

- 2 tsp. butter (unsalted)
- 6 tsp. butter (peanut)
- 3 tsp. of flavored jelly
- 2 pieces of bread

Directions:

1. Put the peanut butter evenly on one bread. Add the layer of jelly.

2. Butter the outside of the pieces of bread.

3. Add the sandwich to a frying pan and toast both sides.

Nutrition: Calories: 300 Fat: 7g Carbs: 49g Protein: 8g Sodium: 460mg Potassium: 222mg Phosphorus: 80mg

10. Grilled Onion and Pepper Jack Grilled Cheese Sandwich

Preparation Time: 5 minutes

Cooking Time: 5 minutes

Servings: 2

Ingredients:

- 1 tsp. of oil (olive)
- 6 tsp. of whipped cream cheese
- 1/2 of a medium onion
- 2 ounces of pepper jack cheese
- 4 slices of rye bread
- 2 tsp. of unsalted butter

Directions:

1. Set out the butter so that it becomes soft. Slice up the onion into thin slices.

2. Sauté onion slices. Continue to stir until cooked. Remove and put it to the side.

3. Spread one tablespoon of the whipped cream cheese on two of the slices of bread.

4. Then add grilled onions and cheese to each slice. Then top using the other two bread slices.

5. Spread the softened butter on the outside of the slices of bread.

6. Use the skillet to toast the sandwiches until lightly brown and the cheese is melted.

Nutrition: Calories: 350 Fat: 18g Carbs: 34g Protein: 13g Sodium: 589mg Potassium: 184mg Phosphorus: 226mg

11. Aromatic Carrot Cream

Preparation Time: 15 minutes

Cooking Time: 25 minutes

Servings: 4

Ingredients:

- 1 tablespoon olive oil
- ½ sweet onion, chopped
- 2 teaspoons fresh ginger, peeled and grated
- 1 teaspoon fresh garlic, minced
- 4 cups water
- 3 carrots, chopped
- 1 teaspoon ground turmeric
- ½ cup coconut almond milk

Directions:

1. Heat the olive oil into a big pan over medium-high heat.
2. Add the onion, garlic and ginger. Softly cook for about 3 minutes until softened.
3. Include the water, turmeric and the carrots. Softly cook for about 20 minutes (until the carrots are softened).
4. Blend the soup adding coconut almond milk until creamy.
5. Serve and enjoy!

Nutrition: Calories 112 Fat 10 g Cholesterol 0 mg Carbohydrates 8 g Sugar 5 g Fiber 2 g Protein 2 g Sodium 35 mg Calcium 32 mg Phosphorus 59 mg Potassium 241 mg

DINNER

12. Cabbage and Beef Fry

Preparation Time: 5 minutes

Cooking Time: 15 minutes

Servings: 4

Ingredients:

- 1 pound beef, ground
- 1/2 pound bacon
- 1 onion
- 1 garlic cloves, minced
- 1/2 head cabbage
- Salt and pepper to taste

Directions:

1. Take a skillet and place it over medium heat
2. Add chopped bacon, beef and onion until slightly browned
3. Transfer to a bowl and keep it covered
4. Add minced garlic and cabbage to the skillet and cook until slightly browned
5. Return the ground beef mixture to the skillet and simmer for 3-5 minutes over low heat
6. Serve and enjoy!

Nutrition: Calories: 360 kcal Total Fat: 22 g Saturated Fat: 0 g Cholesterol: 0 mg Sodium: 0 mg Total Carbs: 5 g

13. California Pork Chops

Preparation Time: 10 minutes

Cooking Time: 10 minutes

Servings: 2

Ingredients:

- 1 tbsp. fresh cilantro, chopped
- 1/2 cup chives, chopped
- 2 large green bell peppers, chopped
- 1 lb. 1" thick boneless pork chops
- 1 tbsp. fresh lime juice
- 2 cups cooked rice
- 1/8 tsp. dried oregano leaves
- 1/4 tsp. ground black pepper
- 1/4 tsp. ground cumin
- 1 tbsp. butter
- 1 lime

Directions:

1. Start by seasoning the pork chops with lime juice and cilantro.
2. Place them in a shallow dish.
3. Toss the chives with pepper, cumin, butter, oregano and rice in a bowl.

4. Stuff the bell peppers with this mixture and place them around the pork chops.

5. Cover the chop and bell peppers with a foil sheet and bake them for 10 minutes in the oven at 375 degrees f.

6. Serve warm.

Nutrition: Calories: 265 kcal Total Fat: 15 g Saturated Fat: 0 g Cholesterol: 86 mg Sodium: 70 mg Total Carbs: 24 g Fiber: 1 g Sugar: 0 g Protein: 34 g

14. Caribbean Turkey Curry

Preparation Time: 10 minutes

Cooking Time: 1 hour an 30 minutes

Servings: 6

Ingredients:

- 3 1/2 lbs. turkey breast, with skin
- 1/4 cup butter, melted
- 1/4 cup honey
- 1 tbsp. mustard
- 2 tsp. curry powder
- 1 tsp. garlic powder

Directions:

1. Place the turkey breast in a shallow roasting pan.
2. Insert a meat thermometer to monitor the temperature.
3. Bake the turkey for 1.5 hours at 350 degrees f until its internal temperature reaches 170 degrees f.
4. Meanwhile, thoroughly mix honey, butter, curry powder, garlic powder, and mustard in a bowl.
5. Glaze the cooked turkey with this mixture liberally.
6. Let it sit for 15 minutes for absorption.
7. Slice and serve.

Nutrition: Calories: 275 kcal Total Fat: 13 g Saturated Fat: 0 g Cholesterol: 82 mg Sodium: 122 mg Total Carbs: 90 g

MAIN DISHES

15. White and Green Quiche

Preparation Time: 10 minutes

Cooking Time: 40 minutes

Servings: 3

Ingredients:

- 3 cups of fresh spinach, chopped
- 15 large free-range eggs
- 3 cloves of garlic, minced
- 5 white mushrooms, sliced
- 1 small sized onion, finely chopped
- 1 ½ teaspoon of baking powder
- Ground black pepper to taste
- 1 ½ cups of coconut almond milk
- Ghee, as required to grease the dish
- Sea salt to taste

Directions:

1. Set the oven to 350°F.
2. Get a baking dish then grease it with the organic ghee.
3. Break all the eggs in a huge bowl then whisk well.
4. Stir in coconut almond milk. Beat well
5. While you are whisking the eggs, start adding the remaining ingredients in it.

6. When all the ingredients are thoroughly blended, pour all of it into the prepared baking dish.
7. Bake for at least 40 minutes, up to the quiche is set in the middle.
8. Enjoy!

Nutrition: Calories: 608 kcal Protein: 20.28 g Fat: 53.42 g Carbohydrates: 16.88 g

16. Beef Breakfast Casserole

Preparation Time: 10 minutes

Cooking Time: 30 minutes

Servings: 5

Ingredients:

- 1 pound of ground beef, cooked
- 10 eggs
- ½ cup Pico de Gallo
- 1 cup baby spinach
- ¼ cup sliced black capers
- Freshly ground black pepper

Directions:

1. Preheat oven to 350 degrees Fahrenheit. Prepare a 9" glass pie plate with non-stick spray.
2. Whisk the eggs until frothy. Season with salt and pepper.
3. Layer the cooked ground beef, Pico de Gallo, and spinach in the pie plate.
4. Slowly pour the eggs over the top.
5. Top with black capers.
6. Bake for at least 30 minutes, until firm in the middle.
7. Slice into 5 pieces and serve.

Nutrition: Calories: 479 kcal Protein: 43.54 g Fat: 30.59 g Carbohydrates: 4.65 g

17. Ham and Veggie Frittata Muffins

Preparation Time: 10 minutes

Cooking Time: 25 minutes

Servings: 12

Ingredients:

- 5 ounces thinly sliced ham
- 8 large eggs
- 4 tablespoons coconut oil
- ½ yellow onion, finely diced
- 8 oz. frozen spinach, thawed and drained
- 8 oz. mushrooms, thinly sliced
- 1 cup cherry bell pepper, halved
- ¼ cup coconut almond milk (canned)
- 2 tablespoons coconut flour
- Sea salt and pepper to taste

Directions:

1. Preheat oven to 375 degrees Fahrenheit.
2. In a medium skillet, warm the coconut oil on medium heat. Add the onion and cook until softened.
3. Add the mushrooms, spinach, and cherry bell pepper. Season with salt and pepper. Cook until the mushrooms have softened. About 5 minutes. Remove from heat and set aside.
4. In a huge bowl, beat the eggs together with the coconut almond milk and coconut flour. Stir in the cooled the veggie mixture.

5. Line each cavity of a 12 cavity muffin tin with the thinly sliced ham. Pour the egg mixture into each one and bake for 20 minutes.
6. Remove from oven and allow to cool for about 5 minutes before transferring to a wire rack.
7. To maximize the benefit of a vegetable-rich diet, it's important to eat a variety of colors, and these veggie-packed frittata muffins do just that. The onion, spinach, mushrooms, and cherry bell pepper provide a wide range of vitamins and nutrients and a healthy dose of fiber.

Nutrition: Calories: 125 kcal Protein: 5.96 g Fat: 9.84 g Carbohydrates: 4.48 g

SNACKS

18. Chocolate-Cashew Spread

Preparation time: 10 minutes

Cooking time: 10 minutes

Servings: Makes ½ cup (2 tablespoons per serving)

Ingredients:

- ¼ cup unsalted cashew butter
- 3 tablespoons water
- 1½ tablespoons unsweetened cocoa powder
- 2 teaspoons honey
- 1 teaspoon extra-virgin olive oil
- ½ teaspoon vanilla extract
- Pinch of ground cinnamon
- Pinch of salt

1. Stir together the cashew butter, water, cocoa powder, honey, olive oil, vanilla, cinnamon, and salt in a large bowl until smooth, 2 to 3 minutes.

Nutrition: Calories: 108; Total Fat: 9g; Saturated Fat: 2g; Cholesterol: 0mg; Sodium: 93mg; Carbohydrates: 8g; Fiber: 1g; Added Sugars: 3g; Protein: 2g; Potassium: 92mg; Vitamin K: 5mcg

19. Mango Chiller

Preparation time: 5 minutes

Cooking time: 5 minutes

Servings: 4 (½ cup per serving)

Ingredients:

- 2 cups frozen mango chunks
- ½ cup plain 2% Greek yogurt
- ¼ cup 1% almond milk
- 2 teaspoons honey (optional)

1. Mix the mango and yogurt in a food processor or blender. Add the almond milk, a bit at a time, to get it to soft ice cream consistency.

2. Taste, and add honey if you like. Enjoy immediately.

Nutrition: Calories: 85; Total Fat: 1g; Saturated Fat: 1g; Cholesterol: 4mg; Sodium: 17mg; Carbohydrates: 16g; Fiber: 1g; Added Sugars: 3g; Protein: 4g; Potassium: 197mg; Vitamin K: 3mcg

20. **Blueberry-Ricotta SwirL**

Preparation time: 5 minutes

Cooking time: 5 minutes

Servings: 2

Ingredients:

- ½ cup fresh or frozen blueberries
- ½ cup part-skim ricotta cheese
- 1 teaspoon sugar
- ½ teaspoon lemon zest (optional)

Directions:

1. If using frozen blueberries, warm them in a saucepan over medium heat until they are thawed but not hot.

2. Meanwhile, mix the sugar with the ricotta in a medium bowl.

3. Mix the blueberries into the ricotta, leaving a few out. Taste, and add more sugar if desired. Top with the remaining blueberries and lemon zest (if using).

Nutrition: Calories: 113; Total Fat: 5g; Saturated Fat: 3g; Cholesterol: 19mg; Sodium: 62mg; Carbohydrates: 10g; Fiber: 1g; Added Sugars: 2g; Protein: 7g; Potassium: 98mg; Vitamin K: 7mcg

21. Roasted Broccoli and Cauliflower

Preparation Time: 7 minutes

Cooking Time: 23 minutes

Serving: 6

Ingredients:

- 2 cups broccoli florets
- 2 cups cauliflower florets
- 2 tablespoons olive oil
- 1 tablespoon freshly squeezed lemon juice
- 2 teaspoons Dijon mustard
- ¼ teaspoon garlic powder
- Pinch salt
- 1/8 teaspoon freshly ground black pepper

Direction

1. Preheat the oven to 425°F.
2. On a baking sheet with a lip, combine the broccoli and cauliflower florets in one even layer.
3. In a small bowl, combine the olive oil, lemon juice, mustard, garlic powder, salt, and pepper until well blended and drizzle the mixture over the vegetables. Toss to coat and spread the vegetables out in a single layer again.
4. Roast for 22 minutes. Serve immediately.

Nutrition: 63 Calories 74mg Sodium 39mg Phosphorus 216mg Potassium 2g Protein

22. Herbed Garlic Cauliflower Mash

Preparation Time: 10 minutes

Cooking Time: 20 minutes

Serving: 6

Ingredients:

- 4 cups cauliflower florets
- 4 garlic cloves, peeled
- 4 ounces cream cheese, softened
- ¼ cup unsweetened almond milk
- 2 tablespoons unsalted butter
- Pinch salt
- 2 tablespoons minced fresh chives
- 2 tablespoons chopped flat-leaf parsley
- 1 tablespoon fresh thyme leaves

Direction

1. Boil water at high heat. Add the cauliflower and garlic and cook, stirring occasionally, until the cauliflower is tender, about 8 to 10 minutes.

2. Drain the cauliflower and garlic into a colander in the sink and shake the colander well to remove excess water.

3. Using a paper towel, blot the vegetables to remove any remaining water. Return the florets to the pot and place

over low heat for 1 minute to remove as much water as possible.

4. Mash the florets and garlic with a potato masher until smooth.

5. Beat in the cream cheese, almond milk, butter, salt, chives, parsley, and thyme with a spoon. Serve.

Nutrition: 124 Calories 115mg Sodium 59mg Phosphorus 266mg Potassium 3g Protein

SOUP AND STEW

23. Egg Tuna Salad

Preparation Time: 10 minutes

Cooking Time: 5 minutes

Servings: 6

Ingredients:

- 8 eggs, hard-boiled, peeled and chopped
- 1/8 tsp paprika
- 1 tsp Dijon mustard
- 2 tbsp. mayonnaise
- 1/3 cup yogurt
- 2 tbsp. chives, minced
- 2 tbsp. onion, minced
- 5 oz. tuna, drain
- Pepper
- Salt

Directions:

1. In a large bowl, whisk together mustard, mayonnaise, yogurt, pepper, and salt.
2. Add eggs, chives, onion, and tuna and mix well.
3. Sprinkle with paprika and serve.

Nutrition: Calories 159 Fat 9.6 g Carbohydrates 3 g Sugar 1.9 g Protein 14.6 g Cholesterol 228 mg Phosphorus: 110mg Potassium: 117mg Sodium: 75mg

24. Chicken Vegetable Salad

Preparation Time: 10 minutes

Cooking Time: 10 minutes

Servings: 4

Ingredients:

- 1 1/2 lbs. cooked chicken, cubed
- 1 cup cherry Red bell peppers, halved
- 4 small zucchinis, trimmed and sliced
- 8 oz. green beans, trimmed
- 1 tbsp. olive oil
- 1/2 small onion, sliced
- 2 tbsp. pesto
- Pepper
- Salt

Directions:

1. Add green beans into the boiling water and cook for 2 minutes. Drain well and transfer in large bowl.
2. Add remaining ingredients to the bowl and toss well.
3. Serve and enjoy.

Nutrition: Calories 369 Fat 12.3 g Carbohydrates 11.1 g Sugar 4.9 g Protein 53 g Cholesterol 133 mg Phosphorus: 110mg Potassium: 117mg Sodium: 75mg

25. Protein Packed Shrimp Salad

Preparation Time: 10 minutes

Cooking Time: 10 minutes

Servings: 4

Ingredients:

- 1 lb. shrimp, peeled and deveined
- 1 1/2 tbsp. fresh dill, chopped
- 1 tsp Dijon mustard
- 2 tsp fresh lemon juice
- 2 tbsp. onion, minced
- 1/2 cup celery, diced
- 1/2 cup mayonnaise
- Pepper
- Salt

Directions:

1. Add shrimp in boiling water and cook for 2 minutes. Drain well and transfer in large bowl.

2. Add remaining ingredients into the bowl and mix well.

3. Serve and enjoy.

Nutrition: Calories 258 Fat 11.9 g Carbohydrates 10.4 g Sugar 2.3 g Protein 26.5 g Cholesterol 246 mg Phosphorus: 135mg Potassium: 154mg Sodium: 75mg

26. Pumpkin and Walnut Puree

Preparation Time: 10mins

Cooking Time: 10mins

Serving: 6

Ingredients:

- 100 g walnuts, without shell
- 300 g pumpkin
- 30 ml of almond milk
- 600 ml of water

Directions:

1. Peel the walnuts and pound them with the mortar.
2. Peel the pumpkin and cut into pieces. Place the pumpkin pieces in a plastic bag and place it in the microwave over a high temperature for five minutes.
3. Put the water with the pumpkin and walnuts in the blender and puree.
4. Put everything in a saucepan and cook until mushy over low heat.
5. Slowly pour in the almond milk and stir.

Nutrition: Calories 53, White eggs 2 g, Carbohydrates 4 g, Fat 4 g, Cholesterol 1 mg, Sodium 167 mg, Potassium 201 mg, Calcium 23 mg, Phosphorus 59 mg, Dietary fiber 1.2 g

VEGETABLE

27. Vegetable Green Curry

Preparation Time: 20 minutes

Cooking Time: 20 minutes

Servings: 6

Ingredients:

- 2 tablespoons extra-virgin olive oil
- 1 head broccoli, cut into florets
- 1 bunch asparagus, cut into 2-inch lengths
- 3 tablespoons water
- 2 tablespoons green curry paste
- 1 medium eggplant
- 1/8 teaspoon salt
- 1/8 teaspoon freshly ground black pepper
- 2/3 cup plain whole-almond milk yogurt

Directions:

1. Put olive oil in a large saucepan in a medium heat. Add the broccoli and stir-fry for 5 minutes. Add the asparagus and stir-fry for another 3 minutes.
2. Meanwhile, in a small bowl, combine the water with the green curry paste.
3. Add the eggplant, curry-water mixture, salt, and pepper. Stir-fry or until vegetables are all tender.

4. Add the yogurt. Heat through but avoid simmering. Serve.

Nutrition: Calories: 113 Total fat: 6g Saturated fat: 1gSodium: 174mg Phosphorus: 117mg Potassium: 569mg Carbohydrates: 13g Fiber: 6g Protein: 5g Sugar: 7g

28. Zucchini Bowl

Preparation Time: 10 minutes

Cooking Time: 20 minutes

Servings: 4

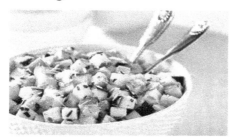

Ingredients:

- 1 onion, chopped
- 3 zucchini, cut into medium chunks
- 2 tablespoons coconut almond milk
- 2 garlic cloves, minced
- 4 cups chicken stock
- 2 tablespoons coconut oil
- Pinch of salt
- Black pepper to taste

Directions:

1. Take a pot and place it over medium heat
2. Add oil and let it heat up
3. Add zucchini, garlic, onion, and stir
4. Cook for 5 minutes
5. Add stock, salt, pepper, and stir
6. Bring to a boil and lower down the heat
7. Simmer for 20 minutes.

8. Remove heat and add coconut almond milk
9. Use an immersion blender until smooth
10. Ladle into soup bowls and serve
11. Enjoy!

Nutrition: Calories: 160 Fat: 2g Carbohydrates: 4g Protein: 7g

29. Nice Coconut Haddock

Preparation Time: 10 minutes

Cooking Time: 12 minutes

Servings: 3

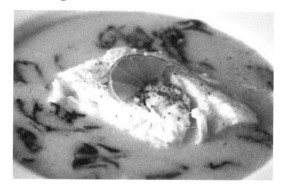

Ingredients:

- 4 haddock fillets, 5 ounces each, boneless
- 2 tablespoons coconut oil, melted
- 1 cup coconut, shredded and unsweetened
- ¼ cup hazelnuts, ground
- Salt to taste

Directions:

1. Preheat your oven to 400 °F
2. Line a baking sheet with parchment paper
3. Keep it on the side
4. Pat fish fillets with a paper towel and season with salt
5. Take a bowl and stir in hazelnuts and shredded coconut
6. Drag fish fillets through the coconut mix until both sides are coated well

7. Transfer to a baking dish
8. Brush with coconut oil
9. Bake for about 12 minutes until flaky
10. Serve and enjoy!

Nutrition: Calories: 299 Fat: 24g Carbohydrates: 1g Protein: 20g

SIDE DISHES

30. Cauliflower and Leeks

Preparation Time: 10 minutes

Cooking Time: 20 minutes

Servings: 4

Ingredients:

- 1 and ½ cups leeks, chopped
- 1 and ½ cups cauliflower florets
- 2 garlic cloves, minced
- 1 and ½ cups artichoke hearts
- 2 tablespoons coconut oil, melted
- Black pepper to taste

Directions:

1. Heat up a pan with the oil over medium-high heat, add garlic, leeks, cauliflower florets and artichoke hearts, stir and cook for 20 minutes.

2. Add black pepper, stir, divide between plates and serve.

3. Enjoy!

Nutrition: Calories 192, fat 6,9, fiber 8,2, carbs 35,1, protein 5,1 Phosphorus: 110mg Potassium: 117mg Sodium: 75mg

31. Eggplant and Mushroom Sauté

Preparation Time: 10 minutes

Cooking Time: 30 minutes

Servings: 4

Ingredients:

- 2 pounds oyster mushrooms, chopped
- 6 ounces shallots, peeled, chopped
- 1 yellow onion, chopped
- 2 eggplants, cubed
- 3 celery stalks, chopped
- 1 tablespoon parsley, chopped
- A pinch of sea salt
- Black pepper to taste
- 1 tablespoon savory, dried
- 3 tablespoons coconut oil, melted

Directions:

1. Heat up a pan with the oil over medium high heat, add onion, stir and cook for 4 minutes.
2. Add shallots, stir and cook for 4 more minutes.
3. Add eggplant pieces, mushrooms, celery, savory and black pepper to taste, stir and cook for 15 minutes.
4. Add parsley, stir again, cook for a couple more minutes, divide between plates and serve.

5. Enjoy!

Nutrition: calories 1013, fat 10,9, fiber 35,5, carbs 156,5, protein 69,1 Phosphorus: 210mg Potassium: 217mg Sodium: 105mg

SALAD

32. Tortellini salad

Preparation time: 5 minutes

Cooking time: 10 minutes

Servings: 4 servings

Ingredients:

- 200g tortellini with meat filling
- 100g red peppers
- 1 tomato
- 1 clove of garlic
- Salt pepper
- fresh basil, some leaves
- 3 tbsp. rapeseed oil
- 1 tbsp. white wine vinegar

Directions:

1. Cook the tortellini in salted water according to the instructions on the packet and drain.

2. Finely dice the pepper and garlic and sweat in the rapeseed oil. Add the vinegar and spices and pour over the tortellini. Cut the tomato into small pieces and mix in. mix with the fresh basil and season to taste.

Nutrition: Energy: 161kcal, Protein: 4g, Fat: 9g, Carbohydrates: 18g, Dietary fibbers: 3g, Potassium: 173mg, Phosphate: 80mg

33. Baked Fennel & Garlic Sea Bass

Preparation Time: 5 minutes

Cooking Time: 15 minutes

Servings: 2

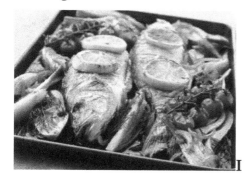

Ingredients:

- 1 lemon
- ½ sliced fennel bulb
- 6 oz. sea bass fillets
- 1 tsp black pepper
- 2 garlic cloves

Directions:

1. Preheat the oven to 375°F. Sprinkle black pepper over the Sea Bass. Slice the fennel bulb and garlic cloves. Add 1 salmon fillet and half the fennel and garlic to one sheet of baking paper or tin foil.

2. Squeeze in 1/2 lemon juices. Repeat for the other fillet. Fold and add to the oven for 12-15 minutes or until fish is thoroughly cooked through.
3. Meanwhile, add boiling water to your couscous, cover, and allow to steam. Serve with your choice of rice or salad.

Nutrition: Calories 221 Protein 14 g Carbs 3 g Fat 2 g Sodium 119 mg Potassium 398 mg Phosphorus 149 mg

34. Lemon, Garlic, Cilantro Tuna and Rice

Preparation Time: 5 minutes

Cooking Time: 0 minutes

Servings: 2

Ingredients:

- ½ cup arugula
- 1 tbsp. extra virgin olive oil
- 1 cup cooked rice
- 1 tsp black pepper
- ¼ finely diced red onion
- 1 juiced lemon
- 3 oz. canned tuna
- 2 tbsp. Chopped fresh cilantro

Directions:

1. Mix the olive oil, pepper, cilantro, and red onion in a bowl. Stir in the tuna, cover, then serve with the cooked rice and arugula!

Nutrition: Calories 221 Protein 11 g Carbs 26 g Fat 7 g Sodium 143 mg Potassium 197 mg Phosphorus 182 mg

35. Cod & Green Bean Risotto

Preparation Time: 4 minutes

Cooking Time: 40 minutes

Servings: 2

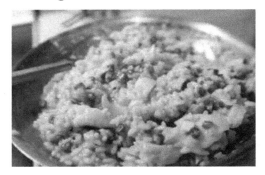

Ingredients:

- ½ cup arugula
- 1 finely diced white onion
- 4 oz. cod fillet
- 1 cup white rice
- 2 lemon wedges
- 1 cup boiling water
- ¼ tsp. black pepper
- 1 cup low-sodium chicken broth
- 1 tbsp. extra virgin olive oil
- ½ cup green beans

Directions:

1. Warm-up oil in a large pan on medium heat. Sauté the chopped onion for 5 minutes until soft before adding in the rice and stirring for 1-2 minutes.

2. Combine the broth with boiling water. Add half of the liquid to the pan and stir. Slowly add the rest of the liquid while continuously stirring for up to 20-30 minutes.
3. Stir in the green beans to the risotto. Place the fish on top of the rice, cover, and steam for 10 minutes.
4. Use your fork to break up the fish fillets and stir into the rice. Sprinkle with freshly ground pepper to serve and a squeeze of fresh lemon. Serve with the lemon wedges and the arugula.

Nutrition: Calories 221 Protein 12 g Carbs 29 g Fat 8 g Sodium 398 mg Potassium 347 mg Phosphorus 241 mg

36. Coconut Cream Shrimp

Preparation Time: 10 minutes

Cooking Time: 20 minutes

Servings: 2

Ingredients:

- 1 tbsp. coconut cream
- ½ tsp. lime juice
- ¼ tsp. black pepper
- 1 tbsp. parsley
- 1 lb. cooked, peeled and deveined shrimp
- ¼ tsp. chopped jalapeno

Directions:

1. In a bowl, mix the shrimp while using cream, jalapeno, lime juice, parsley and black pepper, toss, divide into small bowls and serve.

2. Enjoy!

Nutrition: Calories: 183, Fat: 5 g, Carbs: 12 g, Protein: 8 g, Sugars: 0.9 g, Sodium: 474.9 mg

37. Simple Cinnamon Salmon

Preparation Time: 10 minutes

Cooking Time: 10 minutes

Servings: 2

Ingredients:

- 1 tbsp. organic essential olive oil
- Black pepper
- 1 tbsp. cinnamon powder
- 2 de-boned salmon fillets

Directions:

1. Heat up a pan with the oil over medium heat, add pepper and cinnamon and stir well.

2. Add salmon, skin side up, cook for 5 minutes on both sides, divide between plates and serve by using a side salad.

3. Enjoy!

Nutrition: Calories: 220, Fat: 8 g, Carbs: 11 g, Protein: 8 g, Sugars: 9.3 g, Sodium: 250.5 mg

38. Chicken with Asian Vegetables

Preparation Time: 10 Minutes

Cooking Time: 20 Minutes

Servings: 8

Ingredients:

- 2 tablespoons canola oil
- 6 boneless chicken breasts
- 1 cup low-sodium chicken broth
- 3 tablespoons reduced-sodium soy sauce
- 1/4 teaspoon crushed red pepper flakes
- 1 garlic clove, crushed
- 1 can (8ounces) water chestnuts, sliced and rinsed (optional)
- 1/2 cup sliced green onions
- 1 cup chopped red or green bell pepper
- 1 cup chopped celery
- 1/4 cup cornstarch
- 1/3 cup water
- 3 cups cooked white rice
- 1/2 large chicken breast for 1 chicken thigh

Directions:

1. Warm oil in a skillet and dark-colored chicken on all sides.

2. Add chicken to a slow cooker with the remainder of the fixings aside from cornstarch and water.

3. Spread and cook on LOW for 6 to 8hours

4. Following 6-8 hours, independently blend cornstarch and cold water until smooth. Gradually include into the moderate cooker.

5. At that point turn on high for about 15mins until thickened. Don't close the top on the moderate cooker to enable steam to leave.

6. Serve Asian blend over rice.

Nutrition: Calories 415, Fat 20g, Protein 20g, Carbohydrates 36g

39. Chicken and Veggie Soup

Preparation Time: 15 Minutes

Cooking Time: 25 Minutes

Servings: 8

Ingredients:

- 4 cups cooked and chopped chicken
- 7 cups reduced-sodium chicken broth
- 1-pound frozen white corn
- 1 medium onion diced
- 4 cloves garlic minced
- 2 carrots peeled and diced
- 2 celery stalks chopped
- 2 teaspoons oregano
- 2 teaspoon curry powder
- 1/2 teaspoon black pepper

Directions:

1. Include all fixings into the moderate cooker.
2. Cook on LOW for 8 hours
3. Serve over cooked white rice.

Nutrition: Calories 220, Fat7g, Protein 24g, Carbohydrates 19g

40. **Turkey Sausages**

Preparation Time: 10 Minutes

Cooking Time: 10 Minutes

Servings: 2

Ingredients:

- 1/4 teaspoon salt
- 1/8 teaspoon garlic powder
- 1/8 teaspoon onion powder
- 1 teaspoon fennel seed
- 1 pound 7% fat ground turkey

Directions:

1. Press the fennel seed and in a small cup put together turkey with fennel seed, garlic, and onion powder, and salt.
2. Cover the bowl and refrigerate overnight.
3. Prepare the turkey with seasoning into different portions with a circle form and press them into patties ready to be cooked.
4. Cook at medium heat until browned.
5. Cook it for 1 to 2 minutes per side and serve them hot. Enjoy!

Nutrition: Calories 55, Protein 7 g, Sodium 70 mg, Potassium 105 mg, Phosphorus 75 mg

MEAT RECIPES

41. Sticky Pulled Beef Open Sandwiches

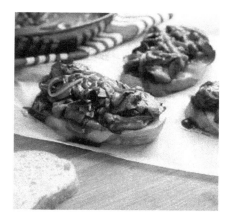

Preparation Time: 15 minutes

Cooking Time: 5 hours

Servings: 5

Ingredients:

- ½ cup of green onion, sliced
- 2 garlic cloves
- 2 tablespoons of fresh parsley
- 2 large carrots
- 7ounce of flat-cut beef brisket, whole
- 1 tablespoon of smoked paprika
- 1 teaspoon dried parsley
- 1 teaspoon of brown sugar
- ½ teaspoon of black pepper
- 2 tablespoon of olive oil

- ¼ cup of red wine
- 8 tablespoon of cider vinegar
- 3 cups of water
- 5 slices white bread
- 1 cup of arugula to garnish

Directions:

1. Finely chop the green onion, garlic, and fresh parsley. Grate the carrot. Put the beef in to roast in a slow cooker.
2. Add the chopped onion, garlic, and remaining ingredients, leaving the rolls, fresh parsley, and arugula to one side. Stir in the slow cooker to combine.
3. Cover and cook on low within 8 1/2 to 10 hours or on high for 4 to 5 hours until tender. Remove the meat from the slow cooker. Shred the meat using two forks.
4. Return the meat to the broth to keep it warm until ready to serve. Lightly toast the bread and top with shredded beef, arugula, fresh parsley, and ½ spoon of the broth. Serve.

Nutrition: Calories: 273 Protein: 15g Carbohydrates: 20g Fat: 11g Sodium: 308mg Potassium: 399mg Phosphorus: 159mg

42. Herby Beef Stroganoff and Fluffy Rice

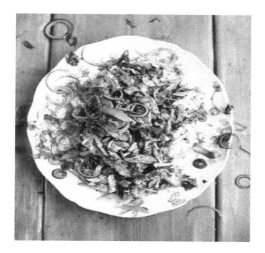

Preparation Time: 15 minutes

Cooking Time: 5 hours

Servings: 6

Ingredients:

- ½ cup onion
- 2 garlic cloves
- 9ounce of flat-cut beef brisket, cut into 1" cubes
- ½ cup of reduced-sodium beef stock
- 1/3 cup red wine
- ½ teaspoon dried oregano
- ¼ teaspoon freshly ground black pepper
- ½ teaspoon dried thyme
- ½ teaspoon of saffron
- ½ cup almond milk (unenriched)
- ¼ cup all-purpose flour
- 1 cup of water

- 2 ½ cups of white rice

Directions:

1. Dice the onion, then mince the garlic cloves. Mix the beef, stock, wine, onion, garlic, oregano, pepper, thyme, and saffron in your slow cooker.
2. Cover and cook on high within 4-5 hours. Combine the almond milk, flour, and water. Whisk together until smooth.
3. Add the flour mixture to the slow cooker. Cook for another 15 to 25 minutes until the stroganoff is thick.
4. Cook the rice using the package instructions, leaving out the salt. Drain off the excess water. Serve the stroganoff over the rice.

Nutrition: Calories: 241 Protein: 15g Carbohydrates: 29g Fat: 5g Sodium: 182mg Potassium: 206mg Phosphorus: 151mg

BROTHS, CONDIMENT AND SEASONING

43. Dried Herb Rub

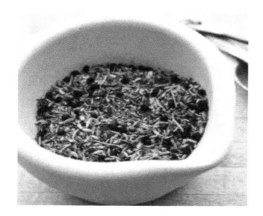

Preparation Time: 15 minutes

Cooking Time: 0 minutes

Servings: 1/3 cup

Ingredients:

- 1 tablespoon dried thyme
- 1 tablespoon dried oregano
- 1 tablespoon dried parsley
- 2 teaspoons dried basil
- 2 teaspoons ground coriander
- 2 teaspoons onion powder
- 1 teaspoon ground cumin
- 1 teaspoon garlic powder

- 1 teaspoon paprika
- ½ teaspoon cayenne pepper

Directions:

1. Put the thyme, oregano, parsley, basil, coriander, onion powder, cumin, garlic powder, paprika, and cayenne pepper in a blender, and pulse until the ingredients are ground and well combined. Transfer the rub to a small container with a lid. Store in a cool, dry area for up to 6 months.

Nutrition: Calories: 3 Fat: 0g Carbohydrates: 1g Phosphorus: 3mg Potassium: 16mg Sodium: 1mg Protein: 0g

44. Mediterranean Seasoning

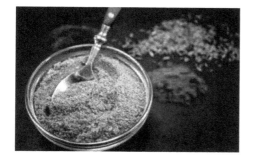

Preparation Time: 15 minutes

Cooking Time: 0 minutes

Servings: 1

Ingredients:

- 2 tablespoons dried oregano
- 1 tablespoon dried thyme
- 2 teaspoons dried rosemary, chopped finely or crushed
- 2 teaspoons dried basil
- 1 teaspoon dried marjoram
- 1 teaspoon dried parsley flakes

Directions:

1. Mix the oregano, thyme, rosemary, basil, marjoram, and parsley in a small bowl until well combined. Transfer then store.

Nutrition: Calories: 1 Fat: 0g Carbohydrates: 0g Phosphorus: 1mg Potassium: 6mg Sodium: 0mg Protein: 0g

DRINKS AND SMOOTHIES

45. Strawberry Fruit Smoothie

Preparation Time: 10minutes

Cooking Time: 0 minutes

Servings: 1

Ingredients:

- 3/4 cup fresh strawberries
- 1/2 cup liquid pasteurized egg whites
- 1/2 cup ice
- 1 tbsp. sugar

Directions:

1. First, start by putting all the ingredients in a blender jug.
2. Give it a pulse for 30 seconds until blended well.
3. Serve chilled and fresh.

Nutrition: Calories 156 Protein 14 g Fat 0 g Cholesterol 0 mg Potassium 400 mg Phosphorus 49 mg Calcium 29 mg Fiber 2.5 g

46. Watermelon Bliss

Preparation Time: 10minutes

Cooking Time: 0 minutes

Servings: 2

Ingredients:

- 2 cups watermelon
- 1 medium-sized cucumber, peeled and sliced
- 2 mint sprigs, leaves only
- 1 celery stalk
- Squeeze of lime juice

Directions:

1. First, start by putting all the ingredients in a blender jug.
2. Give it a pulse for 30 seconds until blended well.
3. Serve chilled and fresh.

Nutrition: Calories 156 Protein 14 g Fat 0 g Cholesterol 0 mg Potassium 400 mg Calcium 29 mg Fiber 2.5g

47. Strawberry ice cream

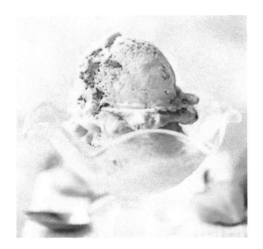

Preparation time: 5 minutes

Cooking time: 5 minutes

Servings: 3 servings

Ingredients:

- Stevia – ½ cup
- Lemon juice – 1 tbsp.
- Non-dairy coffee creamer – ¾ cup
- Strawberries – 10 oz.
- Crushed ice – 1 cup

Directions:

1. Blend everything in a blend until smooth.

2. Freeze until frozen.

3. Serve.

Nutrition: calories: 94.4; fat: 6g; carb: 8.3g; phosphorus: 25mg; potassium: 108mg; sodium: 25mg; protein: 1.3g;

48. Cinnamon custard

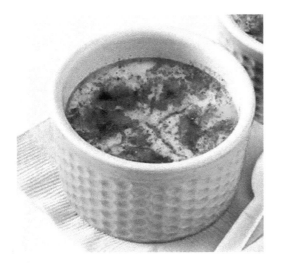

Preparation time: 20 minutes

Cooking time: 1 hour

Servings: 6 servings

Ingredients:

- Unsalted butter, for greasing the ramekins
- Plain rice almond milk – 1 ½ cups
- Eggs – 4
- Granulated sugar – ¼ cup
- Pure vanilla extract – 1 tsp.
- Ground cinnamon – ½ tsp.
- Cinnamon sticks for garnish

Directions:

1. Preheat the oven to 325f.

2. Lightly grease 6 ramekins and place them in a baking dish. Set aside.

3. In a large bowl, whisk together the eggs, rice almond milk, sugar, vanilla, and cinnamon until the mixture is smooth.

4. Pour the mixture through a fine sieve into a pitcher.

5. Evenly divide the custard mixture among the ramekins.

6. Fill the baking dish with hot water, until the water reaches halfway up the ramekins' sides.

7. Bake for 1 hour or until the custards are set and a knife inserted in the center comes out clean.

8. Remove the custards from the oven and take the ramekins out of the water.

9. Cool on the wire racks for 1 hour then chill for 1 hour.

10. garnish with cinnamon sticks and serve.

Nutrition: calories: 110; fat: 4g; carb: 14g; phosphorus: 100mg; potassium: 64mg; sodium: 71mg; protein: 4g;

49. Raspberry brule

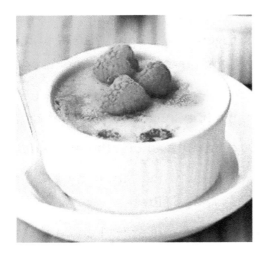

Preparation time: 15 minutes

Cooking time: 1 minute

Servings: 4 servings

Ingredients:

- Light sour cream – ½ cup
- Plain cream cheese – ½ cup
- Brown sugar – ¼ cup, divided
- Ground cinnamon – ¼ tsp.
- Fresh raspberries – 1 cup

Directions:

1. Preheat the oven to broil.

2. In a bowl, beat together the cream cheese, sour cream, 2 tbsp. Brown sugar and cinnamon for 4 minutes or until the mixture is very smooth and fluffy.

3. Evenly divide the raspberries among 4 (4-ounce) ramekins.

4. Spoon the cream cheese mixture over the berries and smooth the tops.

5. Sprinkle ½ tbsp. Brown sugar evenly over each ramekin.

6. Place the ramekins on a baking sheet and broil 4 inches from the heating element until the sugar is caramelized and golden brown.

7. Cool and serve.

Nutrition: calories: 188; fat: 13g; carb: 16g; phosphorus: 60mg; potassium: 158mg; sodium: 132mg; protein

50. Baked egg custard

Preparation time: 15 minutes

Cooking time: 30 minutes

Servings: 4

Ingredients:

- 2 medium eggs, at room temperature
- ¼ cup of semi-skimmed almond milk
- tablespoons of white sugar
- ½ teaspoon of nutmeg
- 1 teaspoon of vanilla extract

Directions:

1 Preheat your oven at 375 f/180c
2 Mix all the ingredients in a mixing bowl and beat with a hand mixer for a few seconds until creamy and uniform.
3 Pour the mixture into lightly greased muffin tins.
4 Bake for 25-30 minutes or until the knife, you place inside, comes out clean.

Nutrition: Calories: 96.56 kcal Carbohydrate: 10.5 g Protein: 3.5 g Sodium: 37.75 mg Potassium: 58.19 mg Phosphorus: 58.76 mg Dietary fiber: 0.06 g Fat: 2.91 g

CPSIA information can be obtained
at www.ICGtesting.com
Printed in the USA
LVHW080027110521
687013LV00002B/170